The Alzheimer's Healing Journey: A Roadmap to Recovery

Louisa Smith

Table of contents

Introduction

Alzheimer's disease is a progressive and debilitating condition that affects millions of people worldwide. It is a complex condition that requires a multifaceted approach to treatment and management. The Alzheimer's Healing Journey: A Roadmap to Recovery is a comprehensive guide to help those who have been diagnosed with Alzheimer's and their caregivers navigate the complex terrain of this disease. The book provides a step-by-step roadmap to recovery that covers a wide range of topics, from understanding the disease and its progression to managing symptoms, engaging in brain-healthy activities, and accessing medical and community resources.

Through this book, readers will learn about evidence-based approaches that can help slow the progression of Alzheimer's, improve cognitive function, and enhance overall quality of life. The roadmap is designed to be practical, accessible, and easy to follow, making it an ideal resource for those who are newly diagnosed or those who have been living with Alzheimer's for some time. Ultimately, The Alzheimer's Healing Journey: A Roadmap to Recovery is a beacon of hope for those affected by this disease, providing valuable insights and guidance that can help them take charge of their health and well-being.

What is Alzheimer's disease?

Alzheimer's disease is a progressive neurodegenerative disorder that affects memory, thinking, and behavior. It is the most common cause of dementia in the elderly population. It is a debilitating condition that can lead to complete loss of independence and functionality. This article will cover the diagnosis and treatment of Alzheimer's disease, including the current understanding of the disease, available diagnostic tools, and treatment options.

Alzheimer's disease is caused by the accumulation of beta-amyloid protein in the brain, which forms plaques, and the accumulation of tau protein, which forms tangles. These plaques and tangles cause damage to the neurons in the brain, leading to their death and the subsequent decline in cognitive and behavioral function.

Early signs and symptoms of Alzheimer's disease

Alzheimer's disease is a progressive, degenerative brain disorder that affects memory, thinking, and behavior. It is the most common form of dementia, accounting for 60-80% of cases. While there is no cure for Alzheimer's disease, early detection and treatment can help manage the symptoms and improve quality of life. In this article, we will explore the early signs and symptoms of Alzheimer's disease.

Memory Loss
One of the most common early signs of Alzheimer's disease is memory loss, particularly short-term memory loss. Forgetting recently learned information, repeating questions or statements, and misplacing objects are all common signs of memory loss in the early

stages of the disease. As the disease progresses, long-term memory can also be affected.

Difficulty with Familiar Tasks

Another early sign of Alzheimer's disease is difficulty performing familiar tasks. This can include forgetting how to cook a meal, operate a household appliance, or use a computer or phone. In the early stages of the disease, individuals may also have difficulty following a recipe or assembling furniture.

Language Problems

Individuals with Alzheimer's disease may also experience difficulty with language. This can include difficulty finding the right words, using the wrong words, or having difficulty understanding what others are saying. As the disease progresses, individuals may have difficulty with reading, writing, and speaking.

Poor Judgment

Another early sign of Alzheimer's disease is poor judgment or decision-making. This can include making poor financial decisions, giving away money to telemarketers or scam artists, or dressing inappropriately for the weather or occasion. In the early stages of the disease, individuals may also have difficulty with personal hygiene or grooming.

Mood Changes
Individuals with Alzheimer's disease may experience mood changes, particularly in the early stages of the disease. This can include becoming more easily agitated, irritable, or suspicious. In some cases, individuals may become more withdrawn or apathetic. Depression is also common in the early stages of Alzheimer's disease.

Withdrawal from Social Activities
Another early sign of Alzheimer's disease is withdrawal from social activities. This can include a loss of interest in hobbies, social activities, or spending time with friends and family. In some cases, individuals may also withdraw from work or other activities they once enjoyed.

Difficulty with Spatial Relationships

Individuals with Alzheimer's disease may also experience difficulty with spatial relationships, particularly in the early stages of the disease. This can include getting lost in familiar places, difficulty judging distances, or difficulty with depth perception.

Confusion and Disorientation
Another common early sign of Alzheimer's disease is confusion and disorientation. This can include difficulty with time, such as not remembering what day it is or getting confused about the time of day. In some cases, individuals may become disoriented in familiar places, such as their own home or neighborhood.

Difficulty with Abstract Thinking
Individuals with Alzheimer's disease may also experience difficulty with abstract thinking, particularly in the early stages of the disease. This can include difficulty with tasks that require planning, organizing, or making decisions.

Alzheimer's disease is a devastating condition that affects millions of people worldwide. While there is no cure for the disease, early detection and treatment can help manage the symptoms and improve quality of life. If you or a loved one is experiencing any of the early signs and symptoms of Alzheimer's disease, it is important to seek medical attention as soon as possible. A healthcare professional can perform a thorough evaluation and determine the best course of action. With the right treatment and support, individuals with Alzheimer's disease can continue to live full and meaningful lives.

Diagnosis and treatment

The diagnosis of Alzheimer's disease is made based on a combination of clinical examination, cognitive testing, and imaging studies. There is no definitive test for Alzheimer's disease, and a diagnosis is usually made after ruling out other possible causes of cognitive decline.

Clinical Examination:

A clinical examination will typically involve a detailed medical history, a physical examination, and a neurological examination. The medical history will include questions about the patient's symptoms, such as memory loss, confusion, and difficulty with activities of daily living. The physical examination will assess the patient's general health and look for signs of neurological impairment, such as weakness or tremors. The neurological examination will assess the patient's cognitive function, including memory, language, and problem-solving abilities.

Cognitive Testing:

Cognitive testing is an essential component of the diagnostic process for Alzheimer's disease. Tests such as the Mini-Mental State Examination (MMSE) or the Montreal Cognitive Assessment (MoCA) are commonly used to assess cognitive function. These tests evaluate memory, attention, language, and visuospatial abilities. The results of cognitive testing can help to determine the severity of cognitive impairment and whether it is consistent with the pattern of cognitive decline seen in Alzheimer's disease.

Imaging Studies:

Imaging studies, such as magnetic resonance imaging (MRI) and positron emission tomography (PET) scans, can help to support a diagnosis of Alzheimer's disease. MRI can detect structural changes in the brain, such as the presence of atrophy or shrinkage in certain areas of the brain. PET scans can detect the accumulation of beta-amyloid protein in the brain.

Treatment of Alzheimer's Disease:

There is currently no cure for Alzheimer's disease, and available treatments focus on managing the symptoms of the disease.

Medications:

Medications are available that can help to improve cognitive function, including acetylcholinesterase inhibitors such as donepezil, galantamine, and rivastigmine. These medications work by increasing the levels of acetylcholine in the brain, a neurotransmitter that is important for memory and learning. Another medication, memantine, is a N-methyl-D-aspartate (NMDA) receptor antagonist that can help to improve cognitive function in some patients.

Non-Pharmacological Interventions:

Non-pharmacological interventions can also be helpful in managing the symptoms of Alzheimer's disease. These may include cognitive stimulation programs, such as puzzles, games, and other activities that can help to maintain cognitive function. Occupational therapy can also be helpful in teaching patients how to manage their daily activities more effectively. Finally, psychotherapy can be useful in helping patients and their families cope with the emotional impact of the disease.

Supportive Care:

Supportive care is an essential component of the management of Alzheimer's disease. This may involve providing assistance with activities of daily living, such as bathing, dressing, and eating. Caregivers may also need support, including respite care, counseling, and education about the disease.

Pharmacological Therapy

There are currently two classes of medications approved by the US Food and Drug Administration (FDA) for the treatment of Alzheimer's disease: cholinesterase inhibitors and N-methyl-D-aspartate (NMDA) receptor antagonists. Cholinesterase inhibitors, such as donepezil, galantamine, and rivastigmine, work by increasing the availability of the neurotransmitter acetylcholine in the brain, which is important for learning and memory. NMDA receptor antagonists, such as memantine, work by modulating the activity of the NMDA receptor, which is involved in learning and memory. These medications can help to improve cognitive function, although their effects are generally modest and may vary from patient to patient.

Non-Pharmacological Therapy:

Non-pharmacological interventions can also be helpful in managing the symptoms of Alzheimer's disease. Cognitive stimulation programs, such as puzzles, games, and other activities that can help to maintain cognitive function, may be useful. Occupational therapy can also be helpful in teaching patients how to manage their daily activities more effectively. Psychotherapy can be useful in helping patients and their families cope with the emotional impact of the disease. Other interventions that may be helpful include physical exercise, music therapy, and art therapy.

Caregiver Support:

Caregiver support is an important aspect of the management of Alzheimer's disease. Caregivers may experience a variety of physical, emotional, and financial challenges as they care for a loved one with Alzheimer's disease. Respite care, which involves providing temporary relief for caregivers, can be helpful in reducing caregiver stress and improving quality of life for both the caregiver and the patient. Caregiver education programs can provide information and training on how to manage the day-to-day care of a patient with Alzheimer's disease, as well as on how to cope with the emotional impact of the disease.

Hospice Care:

As Alzheimer's disease progresses, patients may experience a variety of physical and psychological symptoms, including pain, anxiety, depression, and difficulty with eating and drinking. Hospice care, which is focused on providing comfort and support for patients who are nearing the end of life, can be helpful in managing these symptoms and improving quality of life for patients and their families. Hospice care can be provided in a variety of settings, including the patient's home, a hospice facility, or a nursing home.

Alzheimer's disease is a challenging and complex disorder that requires a comprehensive approach to management. While there is no cure for the disease, a variety of therapies and interventions can help to manage the symptoms of the disease and improve quality of life for patients and their caregivers. Pharmacological therapy, non-pharmacological therapy, caregiver support, and hospice care are all important components of the management of Alzheimer's

disease. As our understanding of the disease
continues to evolve, it is likely that new
therapies and interventions will be developed
that can further improve the lives of patients
and their families

Coping with the diagnosis

Receiving a diagnosis of Alzheimer's disease can be an overwhelming and emotional experience for both the individual and their loved ones. Coping with this diagnosis can be difficult, but it is essential to establish coping mechanisms to ensure the best quality of life for the individual living with Alzheimer's disease and their family. This article will explore how individuals and their families can cope with the emotional impact of an Alzheimer's disease diagnosis, including how to communicate with loved ones and caregivers, and how to make plans for the future.

Understanding Alzheimer's Disease

Alzheimer's disease is a progressive brain disorder that affects memory, thinking, and behavior. The disease gradually destroys brain cells and leads to cognitive impairment, functional decline, and eventually, death. There is no cure for Alzheimer's disease, but there are medications and lifestyle changes that can help manage symptoms and slow the progression of the disease.

It is crucial to communicate your feelings and concerns with loved ones and healthcare professionals. Open communication can help everyone involved in the care process understand the diagnosis and work together to develop a plan for the future. Remember that you are not alone, and there are support groups and resources available to help you cope with the emotional impact of the diagnosis.

Communication with Loved Ones and Caregivers

Communication is key when coping with an Alzheimer's disease diagnosis. It is essential to communicate openly and honestly with loved ones and caregivers to ensure that everyone is on the same page when it comes to care and support. Here are some tips for effective communication:

Be clear and concise: When communicating, try to be clear and concise with your message to avoid confusion.

Listen actively: Listen actively to what others are saying and ask for clarification if needed.

Use nonverbal cues: Nonverbal cues such as facial expressions and body language can help convey your message.

Be patient: Alzheimer's disease can affect an individual's ability to communicate, so it is essential to be patient and understanding.

Use humor: Using humor can help lighten the mood and ease tensions during difficult conversations.

Making Plans for the Future

It is essential to make plans for the future when coping with an Alzheimer's disease diagnosis.

These plans can help ensure that the individual with Alzheimer's disease receives the care and support they need while maintaining their quality of life. Here are some tips for making plans for the future:

Develop a care plan: Work with healthcare professionals to develop a care plan that outlines the individual's needs and preferences.

Choose a caregiver: Choose a caregiver who is reliable, trustworthy, and has experience caring for someone with Alzheimer's disease.

Create a support network: Build a support network of family, friends, and healthcare professionals who can offer assistance and support.

Explore long-term care options: Explore long-term care options such as assisted living facilities and nursing homes, if necessary.

Plan for legal and financial issues: Plan for legal and financial issues such as power of attorney, living wills, and estate planning.

Coping with an Alzheimer's disease diagnosis can be challenging, but it is essential to establish coping mechanisms to ensure the best quality of life for the individual living with Alzheimer's disease and their family. Open communication, support from loved ones and healthcare professionals, and making plans for the future can help ease the emotional impact of the diagnosis and ensure that the individual with Alzheimer's disease receives the care and support they need. Remember that there are resources and

Managing symptoms

Alzheimer's disease is a progressive brain disorder that affects memory, thinking, and behavior. It is the most common cause of dementia, which is a general term used to describe a decline in cognitive function that interferes with daily life. While there is no cure for Alzheimer's disease, there are several ways to manage its symptoms and improve quality of life for both patients and their caregivers.

In this article, we will discuss different ways to manage the symptoms of Alzheimer's disease, including cognitive stimulation and lifestyle changes, as well as the role of medications in treating the disease.

Cognitive Stimulation

Cognitive stimulation is a technique used to help individuals with Alzheimer's disease maintain cognitive function and independence for as long as possible. The aim is to engage patients in activities that challenge their brains and encourage them to think and problem-solve. Some examples of cognitive stimulation activities include:

Memory games: Memory games such as card matching, word games, or crossword puzzles can help improve memory function and prevent cognitive decline.

Music therapy: Music can be a powerful tool in engaging patients with Alzheimer's disease. Listening to music or playing musical instruments can help improve mood, reduce anxiety, and stimulate memory.

Art therapy: Art therapy involves engaging patients in creative activities such as painting, drawing, or sculpture. These activities can improve mood and provide a sense of accomplishment and purpose.

Reading: Reading can help stimulate the brain and improve cognitive function. Patients can read books, newspapers, or magazines, depending on their interests and abilities.

Social activities: Engaging in social activities such as playing games, going out to eat, or attending social events can help improve mood and social interaction. Social interaction can help reduce the risk of depression and cognitive decline.

Lifestyle Changes

In addition to cognitive stimulation, lifestyle changes can also help manage the symptoms of Alzheimer's disease. Some of the lifestyle changes that can help manage the symptoms of Alzheimer's disease include:

Exercise: Regular exercise can help improve cognitive function, reduce anxiety and depression, and improve overall physical health. Even light exercise such as walking can have a significant impact on cognitive function.

Nutrition: A healthy diet can help improve overall health and cognitive function. A diet rich in fruits, vegetables, whole grains, and lean proteins is recommended for patients with Alzheimer's disease.

Sleep: Getting adequate sleep is important for overall health and can help improve cognitive function. Patients with Alzheimer's disease should aim for at least 7-8 hours of sleep per night.

Stress management: Stress can worsen symptoms of Alzheimer's disease. Patients should learn stress management techniques such as deep breathing, meditation, or yoga.

Routine: Establishing a routine can help patients with Alzheimer's disease feel more in control and reduce confusion. This routine can include daily activities such as meal times, exercise, and social interaction.

Medications

While there is no cure for Alzheimer's disease, there are medications available that can help manage its symptoms. These medications work by regulating the levels of neurotransmitters in the brain, which can improve cognitive function and reduce symptoms such as memory loss, confusion, and agitation.

Some of the medications commonly used to treat Alzheimer's disease include:

Cholinesterase inhibitors: These medications work by increasing the levels of acetylcholine in the brain, which is a neurotransmitter that plays a key role in learning and memory. Examples of cholinesterase inhibitors include donepezil, rivastigmine, and galantamine.

Memantine: Memantine is a medication that works by regulating the levels of glutamate in the brain, which is a neurotransmitter that can cause damage to the brain in excess amounts. Memantine can help improve cognitive function and reduce symptoms such as confusion and agitation.

Lifestyle changes are an important part of managing the symptoms of Alzheimer's disease, but they are not always enough on their own. Medications can be a valuable tool in managing symptoms and improving quality of life for patients with Alzheimer's disease.

It is important to note that these medications do not cure Alzheimer's disease, and their effects are temporary. They can help manage symptoms for a period of time, but eventually, the disease will continue to progress. Medications may also have side effects, and their effectiveness can vary from person to person.

It is essential that patients and caregivers work closely with their healthcare providers to monitor the effects of medications and make any necessary adjustments to treatment plans. Patients with Alzheimer's disease should also have regular check-ups with their healthcare providers to monitor their cognitive function, overall health, and the progression of the disease.

Alzheimer's disease is a challenging and progressive brain disorder that affects millions of people worldwide. While there is no cure for the disease, there are several ways to manage its symptoms and improve quality of life for both patients and their caregivers.

Cognitive stimulation, lifestyle changes, and medications are all valuable tools in managing the symptoms of Alzheimer's disease. Cognitive stimulation activities such as memory games, music therapy, and art therapy can help maintain cognitive function and improve mood. Lifestyle changes such as exercise, nutrition, and stress management can help improve overall health and reduce the risk of cognitive decline. Medications such as cholinesterase inhibitors and memantine can help manage symptoms and improve cognitive function, but they are not a cure and can have side effects.

Managing the symptoms of Alzheimer's disease requires a comprehensive approach that takes into account the unique needs and abilities of each patient. It is essential that patients and caregivers work closely with their healthcare providers to develop a customized treatment plan that addresses their individual needs and goals. With the right combination of cognitive stimulation, lifestyle changes, and medications, patients with Alzheimer's disease can maintain their independence and quality of life for as long as possible.

Living with Alzheimer's disease

Individuals with Alzheimer's disease experience a wide range of symptoms, which can include memory loss, disorientation, confusion, mood swings, and difficulty with communication. As the disease progresses, these symptoms can become more severe, and individuals may experience difficulty with basic tasks such as eating, bathing, and dressing themselves. People with Alzheimer's disease may also become increasingly dependent on others for their care and support.

One of the most challenging aspects of living with Alzheimer's disease is the progressive loss of memory. This can be particularly distressing for individuals who are used to being independent and self-reliant. They may struggle to remember the names of family members and friends, forget important events or appointments, and have difficulty navigating familiar environments. As a result, they may become isolated and withdrawn, which can lead to feelings of loneliness and depression.

Another common challenge faced by individuals with Alzheimer's disease is communication. As the disease progresses, individuals may struggle to express themselves and to understand others. They may have difficulty finding the right words or organizing their thoughts, which can lead to frustration and anxiety. They may also misinterpret social cues or become agitated in response to changes in their environment or routine.

In addition to these challenges, individuals with Alzheimer's disease may also experience physical symptoms, such as loss of appetite, weight loss, and difficulty with mobility. They may also be at increased risk of falls and other accidents, which can lead to serious injuries.

Despite these challenges, many individuals with Alzheimer's disease are able to maintain a high quality of life through the use of coping strategies and support from their loved ones. One effective strategy is to maintain a regular routine and a familiar environment. This can help individuals with Alzheimer's disease to feel more secure and in control, which can reduce feelings of anxiety and confusion.

Another important coping strategy is to engage in activities that are stimulating and enjoyable. This can include hobbies such as gardening, painting, or listening to music, which can help to maintain cognitive function and improve mood. It is also important for individuals with Alzheimer's disease to stay socially engaged and to maintain relationships with family and friends.

For some individuals with Alzheimer's disease, medication can be an effective way to manage symptoms such as memory loss and confusion. There are also non-pharmacological interventions that can help to improve cognitive function and reduce behavioral symptoms.

These can include cognitive stimulation therapy, which involves structured activities designed to improve memory and problem-solving skills, and behavioral interventions such as relaxation techniques and stress management.

For individuals with more advanced Alzheimer's disease, it may be necessary to receive care in a specialized dementia care facility. These facilities offer a range of services designed to support individuals with Alzheimer's disease and their families, including assistance with daily activities, medication management, and social and recreational programs.

Living with Alzheimer's disease can be challenging and stressful, both for individuals with the disease and for their loved ones. However, with the right support and coping strategies, it is possible to maintain a high quality of life and to continue to enjoy meaningful relationships and activities. By remaining informed and involved in the management of the disease, individuals with

Alzheimer's disease and their families can work together to promote independence, dignity, and well-being

Prevention and risk factors

Alzheimer's disease is a progressive neurodegenerative disorder that affects memory, thinking, and behavior. It is the most common cause of dementia among older adults, and its prevalence is expected to rise as the population ages. While there is no cure for Alzheimer's disease, there are steps that individuals can take to reduce their risk of developing the disease or delay its onset. In this article, we will explore the risk factors associated with Alzheimer's disease and discuss how individuals can reduce their risk of developing the disease.

Risk factors for Alzheimer's disease

While the exact cause of Alzheimer's disease is unknown, researchers have identified several risk factors that may contribute to its development. Some of these risk factors cannot be changed, such as age, genetics, and family history, while others can be modified through lifestyle changes.

Age

Age is the most significant risk factor for Alzheimer's disease. The risk of developing the disease doubles every five years after the age of 65. By the age of 85, nearly one in three people have Alzheimer's disease. While aging is inevitable, individuals can take steps to reduce their risk of developing the disease through healthy lifestyle choices.

Genetics

Family history of Alzheimer's disease is also a significant risk factor. If a parent or sibling has Alzheimer's disease, an individual's risk of developing the disease is higher. However, not all cases of Alzheimer's disease are hereditary, and individuals without a family history can still develop the disease. Researchers have identified several genes associated with Alzheimer's disease, but these genetic factors are not a guarantee that an individual will develop the disease.

Lifestyle factors

There are several lifestyle factors that may increase the risk of developing Alzheimer's disease, including:

Poor diet: A diet high in saturated and trans fats and low in fruits, vegetables, and whole grains may increase the risk of developing Alzheimer's disease.
Lack of physical activity: Physical inactivity may increase the risk of developing Alzheimer's disease. Regular exercise can help maintain a healthy weight and improve cardiovascular health, which may reduce the risk of developing the disease.
Smoking: Smoking is a significant risk factor for a variety of health problems, including Alzheimer's disease.

Chronic stress: Chronic stress may increase the risk of developing Alzheimer's disease. Managing stress through relaxation techniques, such as meditation and deep breathing, may help reduce the risk.

Sleep disturbances: Poor sleep quality may increase the risk of developing Alzheimer's disease. Maintaining good sleep hygiene, such as going to bed and waking up at the same time each day, may help reduce the risk.

Medical conditions

Several medical conditions may increase the risk of developing Alzheimer's disease, including:

Cardiovascular disease: High blood pressure, high cholesterol, and other cardiovascular conditions may increase the risk of developing Alzheimer's disease.

Diabetes: Type 2 diabetes may increase the risk of developing Alzheimer's disease. Maintaining good blood sugar control may help reduce the risk.

Traumatic brain injury: A history of traumatic brain injury may increase the risk of developing Alzheimer's disease.

Depression: Depression may increase the risk of developing Alzheimer's disease. Treating depression may help reduce the risk.
Reducing the risk of Alzheimer's disease

While some risk factors for Alzheimer's disease, such as age and genetics, cannot be changed, individuals can take steps to reduce their risk of developing the disease. The following are some ways to reduce the risk of Alzheimer's disease:

Maintain a healthy lifestyle

Maintaining a healthy lifestyle is crucial for reducing the risk of Alzheimer's disease. A healthy lifestyle includes:

Eating a healthy diet: A healthy diet should include plenty of fruits, vegetables, whole grains, and lean protein. Avoiding foods high in saturated and trans fats and limiting sugary and processed foods may help reduce the risk of developing Alzheimer's disease

Advocacy and support

Alzheimer's disease is a debilitating and progressive neurological disorder that affects millions of people worldwide. It is the most common cause of dementia and typically affects individuals over the age of 65. As the disease progresses, it can lead to significant cognitive and behavioral changes that impact the individual's ability to perform daily activities, communicate effectively, and maintain social relationships.

Living with Alzheimer's disease can be challenging, both for the individual with the disease and for their family members and caregivers. This is where advocacy and support play a crucial role. Advocacy involves raising awareness about the disease and the challenges faced by individuals living with Alzheimer's disease and their families. Support resources, such as support groups and community resources, can help individuals with Alzheimer's disease and their families navigate the challenges of the disease and maintain a better quality of life.

Advocacy is important because it helps to increase public awareness and understanding of Alzheimer's disease. When more people are aware of the disease and its impact, it can help reduce stigma and promote understanding and empathy towards those living with the disease. Advocacy can also help to raise funds for research into the causes and treatment of Alzheimer's disease, which can lead to better outcomes for those affected by the disease.

There are many resources available to support individuals with Alzheimer's disease and their families. One of the most valuable resources is support groups. Support groups can provide emotional support, practical advice, and a sense of community to individuals and families affected by the disease. Support groups can also provide a safe and confidential space for individuals to share their experiences, ask questions, and receive support from others who understand what they are going through.

Support groups can take many different forms. Some support groups are led by professionals, such as social workers or counselors, while others are led by individuals with personal experience of Alzheimer's disease. Some support groups are held in person, while others are conducted online or over the phone. Support groups may be specific to certain populations, such as caregivers or individuals with early-stage Alzheimer's disease. There are also support groups that are tailored to cultural or linguistic needs.

In addition to support groups, there are many community resources available to support individuals with Alzheimer's disease and their families. These resources may include adult day care programs, respite care services, and home health care services. Adult day care programs can provide a safe and stimulating environment for individuals with Alzheimer's disease, while also giving caregivers a break from their caregiving responsibilities. Respite care services can provide temporary relief for caregivers who need a break from their caregiving duties. Home health care services can provide assistance with activities of daily living, such as bathing, dressing, and medication management.

There are also many resources available online that can provide information and support to individuals and families affected by Alzheimer's disease. The Alzheimer's Association website, for example, provides information about the disease, as well as resources for caregivers and support groups. The Alzheimer's Foundation of America also provides information and support for individuals and families affected by Alzheimer's disease, including an online support group.

It is important to note that support resources may vary depending on where you live. It is important to research what resources are available in your community and to seek out the support that is most appropriate for your needs. Your healthcare provider, social worker, or local

Alzheimer's Association chapter may be able to provide information about local resources.

In conclusion, advocacy and support play a critical role in the lives of individuals and families affected by Alzheimer's disease. Advocacy helps to increase awareness and understanding of the disease, while support resources such as support groups and community resources provide much-needed emotional and practical support to individuals and families affected by the disease. If you or someone you know is living with Alzheimer's disease, it is important to seek out the support and resources that can help you

www.ingramcontent.com/pod-product-compliance
Lightning Source LLC
Chambersburg PA
CBHW061557250726
48657CB00021B/2199